How to Deal with Emotional Trauma in a Relationship

An Ultimate Guide for Defeating Traumatic Environments and the State of Loneliness Capable of Truncating the Original Purpose of Union.

Adegboye S. Aduragbemi

1

How to Deal with Emotional Trauma in a Relationship   1

A FAQ Guide for Defeating Emotional Traumatic Environments and the State of Loneliness

Capable of Truncating the Original Purpose of Union.   1

INTRODUCTION   4

Chapter One   6

Power of efficiency in marriage   6

    How complications of emotional support may strain solid relationships   6

    The value of open communication and understanding in building a long-lasting relationship   8

Chapter Two   11

    Navigating your relationship emotionally   11

Chapter Three   19

    Handling issues when emotionally depressed   19

Chapter Four   23

    Decision-making in the presence of emotional trials   23

Chapter Five   29

    Securing your relationship from external influence   29

About the Author   33

Acknowledgements   34

INTRODUCTION

Marriage is a haven where hearts meet, minds connect, and souls entwine—it's more than just the joining of two people. As a couple navigates the highs and lows of life together, giving and receiving emotional support becomes crucial during the holy journey of matrimony. However, in the middle of everyday life's complications, concerns about providing, obtaining, and maintaining emotional support within the boundaries of a marriage frequently surface. "Emotional Support FAQ in Marriage" is a valuable resource for married couples who are looking for guidance, comprehension, and practical tips on how to maintain a kind and understanding relationship.

This book contains a thorough list of frequently asked concerns, thoughtful responses, and professional guidance specific to the subtleties of providing emotional support in a married relationship. With the aim of assisting couples in cultivating a culture of empathy, comprehension, and practical advice, every query is addressed, ranging from handling disagreements and providing solace in trying times to jointly rejoicing in victories.

"Emotional Support FAQ in Marriage" provides a road map for couples to improve their emotional connection, weather life's storms with grace and fortitude, and deepen their emotional connection through realistic tales, real-life events, and evidence-based solutions. Whether you're trying to improve the emotional closeness in your relationship or are dealing with relationship difficulties, this book offers priceless advice and doable strategies to help you build a dependable and caring alliance that endures.

May you find comfort in the experiences of others who have gone before you, inspiration in the knowledge of professionals, and the bravery to accept emotional support and vulnerability as the cornerstones of your marriage as you set out on this path of exploration and discovery.

Together, let's explore the ageless issues, complex details, and wonders of emotional support in marriage.

Chapter One

Power of efficiency in marriage

How complications of emotional support may strain solid relationships

Kate and Alex used to be the definition of a happy couple living in the quiet town of Willowbrook. They fell madly in love when they first met in college and hoped to create a comfortable, loving, and devoted life together. But as they dealt with the difficulties of life, their relationship started to fall apart due to unfulfilled emotional demands and a breakdown in communication.

Kate was a kind social worker who had a great heart and dedicated her life to supporting people emotionally and helping those in need. She expected Alex to provide the same degree of emotional support since she valued connection, empathy, and understanding in her relationships. As a pragmatic engineer with an analytical outlook, Alex found it difficult to communicate his feelings and establish an emotional bond with

Kate; instead, he would frequently turn to problem-solve as a coping mechanism.

Tensions increased as Kate and Alex dealt with life's ups and downs, despite their differences in how they provide emotional support at first. Alex felt overburdened and misinterpreted by Kate's constant need for validation and assurance, and Kate frequently felt ignored and disappointed by Alex's incapacity to connect emotionally. Their once-loving relationship turned into a never-ending spiral of anger, discontent, and frustration.

One evening, their problems with emotional support reached a breaking point when a disagreement about Kate's challenging workday turned into a full-fledged argument. When Kate went to Alex for help because she was feeling weak and in need of consolation, she was treated with annoyance and disinterest. Overwhelmed by Kate's emotional demands, Alex pulled farther inward, unable to offer her the understanding and support she so desperately needed.

As the years went by, Kate and Alex's relationship continued to worsen, with their arguments overshadowing any hint of affection or kinship. In a frantic offer to save their marriage, they attempted communication seminars, couples therapy, and even a trial separation, but it didn't work. Ultimately, they both lamented the loss of the love they had previously experienced when they made the painful decision to separate ways.

Years later, Kate and Alex coincidentally crossed paths once more. They couldn't help but feel a twinge of grief for the love they had lost as they made small talk. They came to the realization that their failure to attend to one another's emotional needs had ruined their relationship, and they wished they had placed a higher priority on mutual support, communication, and empathy from the start.

This narrative shows how problems with emotional support may strain even the most solid relationships, emphasizing the value of open communication, empathy, and understanding in building strong and long-lasting bonds.

The value of open communication and understanding in building a long-lasting relationship

Anna and Jake were two people whose lives in the quiet hamlet of Willowbrook were entwined via the power of emotional support, resulting in a partnership built on empathy, compassion, and a profound comprehension of each other's needs. They first connected at a neighbourhood support group where Jake, a kind volunteer committed to serving others, and Anna, a sympathetic therapist with a focus on mental health, got together to offer consolation and comfort to those in need.

They bonded over their experiences of overcoming adversity and helping others through their problems, which led to their earliest contacts being full of empathy and understanding. While Jake was enthralled with Anna's compassion and her capacity to listen to individuals in need and offer consolation, Anna respected Jake's unshakable dedication to improving the lives of others.

As they spent more time together, Anna and Jake developed a close bond and respect for one another that led to a solid and long-lasting alliance. They were able to support and encourage one another through life's hardships, which gave them strength and comfort as they shared their goals, worries, and dreams.

As they relied on one another for support and found solace and understanding in their common path of recovery and development, their relationship thrived. Since they knew they would be one other's rock in difficult times, Anna and Jake built a loving, safe atmosphere where they could express themselves freely.

As their love grew, Anna and Jake committed themselves to one another by exchanging vows in front of loved ones in a touching ceremony. They accepted their duties as life partners and providers of emotional support, confident that their love and awareness of one another's needs would enable them to overcome any obstacles that may arise.

Years later, Anna and Jake proudly and gratefully reflected on their experience. They were aware that empathy, compassion, and a profound comprehension of one another's emotional needs had served as the cornerstones of their relationship. Their relationship had only gotten closer over time, and they were confident that by sticking by one another through thick and thin, they could conquer any challenge and realize their goals as a couple.

This summary emphasizes the value of empathy, compassion, and understanding in creating a solid and long-lasting partnership by showing how a relationship may be constructed

on a foundation of emotional support.

Chapter Two

Navigating your relationship emotionally

How can we help each other emotionally while our

marriage is going through stressful or challenging times?

Active listening, empathy, and validating one another's feelings

are all part of offering emotional support. Establish a judgment-

free environment where both parties feel comfortable sharing

their feelings and worries in order to foster open

communication. Give your partner your whole attention while

engaging in active listening, and then mirror back what you hear to demonstrate your knowledge. To make your spouse feel supported and understood, give them words of affirmation, encouragement, and validation.

How can we show each other emotional support on a regular basis?

Affirmative statements, simple gestures, and deeds of kindness can all be used to express emotional support. Regularly check in with each other to find out how the other is doing and whether they need assistance with anything. Express your gratitude, encouragement, and admiration for all that your partner has worked hard to achieve. Give hugs, kisses, and cuddles to express your physical affection and assurance.

How should we respond when one partner needs more emotional assistance than the other?

Empathy, tolerance, and comprehension are necessary for managing variations in emotional needs. Acknowledge that every individual has distinct methods of managing stress and expressing feelings, and provide assistance to your spouse in order to meet their specific requirements. Talk honestly with your partner about how you need emotional support yourself and how they can best give it to you. Be prepared to make concessions and come to a compromise that benefits both parties. If necessary, you should also look for extra help from friends, family, or a therapist.

How can we provide emotional support to one another in the face of external difficulties or disputes in our lives?

Problem-solving, empathy, and teamwork are necessary for helping one another through difficulties. As a team, approach the problem, coming up with solutions and encouraging one another along the way. Recognize your partner's sentiments and concerns without passing judgment in order to demonstrate active listening and empathy. To reduce stress and show your support, provide helpful assistance, such as aid with tasks or resources.

How can we resolve conflicts between the capacity of one partner to support the other and their emotional needs?

Communication, compromise, and empathy are necessary for resolving issues in emotional support. Commence by talking about your individual moving needs and how they could interfere with each other's capacity to offer support. Be willing to explore different approaches to fulfilling each other's needs, like asking for help from family, friends, or a therapist. Even if you are unable to give your spouse the help they need, you may still demonstrate empathy by acknowledging and understanding their feelings.

How can we make sure that during our marriage, we continue to provide each other with solid and constant emotional support?

Consistent communication, setting priorities, and work are necessary to maintain strong emotional support. Plan frequent check-ins to talk about how you're both feeling and how you might support each other more effectively. Make time for each other that is emotionally connected and strengthens your relationship a priority. Take the initiative to express to your partner your gratitude, love, and support in both words and deeds. Recall that investing in emotional support is crucial for long-term happiness and fulfilment because it is the foundation of a peaceful and healthy relationship.

After a rift or betrayal in our marriage, how can we mend trust and emotional closeness?

It takes time, effort, and dedication from both couples to re-establish intimacy and trust. Start by discussing the betrayal or breach and how it affects your relationship honestly and openly. Listen to your partner's feelings and concerns with compassion and understanding, and express your regret and want to make amends. Rebuilding trust requires proactive measures like setting limits, being open and accountable, and placing a high value on communication and quality time spent together.

Following a betrayal or loss of trust, how do we mend the emotional bonds and trust in our marriage?

Honesty, openness, and patience are necessary to re-establish emotional connection and trust. Begin by expressing sincere regret for any harm caused and admitting the violation of trust. Commit to honest and open communication, and deal honestly and transparently with any questions or issues. Accept accountability for your actions and collaborate to determine the underlying problems that caused the betrayal of trust. Going ahead, set up explicit guidelines and agreements, and give top priority to consistent acts that show your dedication to re-establishing trust. Recognize that restoring trust requires time and work from both parties and act with patience and compassion.

As we get older together, what are some tactics for preserving emotional closeness and connection in our marriage?

Connectivity, communication, and shared experiences must be given top priority in order to maintain emotional closeness. Plan frequent check-ins to talk about your aims and feelings as a partnership and as individuals. Allocate time for rituals and activities that foster emotional closeness and unity. Engage in empathy and active listening by paying attention to each other's wants and worries with sincere concern and interest. When difficulties or disagreements come up, take the initiative to resolve them and give top priority to coming up with solutions that can eventually deepen your emotional connection.

How can we work with emotional differences in our reactions to conflict or stress in a way that makes our partnership stronger?

Communication, understanding, and empathy are necessary to navigate variations in emotional reactions. Acknowledge that depending on their personality qualities and past experiences, people may have varying coping strategies and emotional triggers. Be curious about the problem and open to learning about each other's emotional lives. Recognize each other's emotions and engage in active listening, even if they are different from your own. Instead of increasing hostility or placing blame, use dispute as a chance to learn more about one another and discover points of agreement.

In order to promote our mental and emotional well-being, how can we include emotional self-care into our everyday routine?

Including emotional self-care is giving mental and emotional health-promoting activities and practices a top priority. It can involve practising mindfulness techniques like meditation or deep breathing exercises, taking up enjoyable and relaxing hobbies or pastimes, journaling to process feelings and think back on experiences, asking friends and family for social support, and establishing boundaries to safeguard your emotional time and energy. Try out various self-care techniques to see which ones are most effective for you, then include them in your daily routine.

Chapter Three

Handling issues when emotionally depressed

How do we handle circumstances where one partner's emotional needs fluctuate over time and need modifying our support methods?

It takes adaptability, communication, and flexibility to navigate shifting emotional requirements. Acknowledge that people's emotional demands might change as a result of a variety of things, including stressful situations, life events, or personal development. Please pay attention to your partner's indications and be honest when discussing how their needs are changing. Be prepared to modify your support-giving strategy as necessary, whether that means checking in more frequently, using alternative channels of communication, or pursuing extra options like counselling or therapy.

In order to allow ourselves to express our emotions and weaknesses in our marriage openly, how can we cultivate an atmosphere of emotional safety and trust?

Establishing an atmosphere of acceptance, empathy, and trust is necessary to promote emotional safety. Engage in active listening and offer nonjudgmental validation for each other's emotions and experiences. Establish a secure environment where both partners can communicate honestly and feel free to share their feelings and vulnerabilities. Pay attention to one another's wants and worries, and give priority to settling disputes in a kind and productive way. Keep in mind that creating an environment of trust and emotional safety requires time and work, but it sets the groundwork for a solid and happy marriage.

What should we do when one spouse finds it difficult to help the other emotionally because of their emotional issues or limitations?

Managing difficulties when offering assistance calls for tolerance, compassion, and understanding between parties. Acknowledge that every individual faces unique emotional challenges and constraints, and treat the circumstance with kindness and understanding. Inspire your spouse to express their feelings and worries, and provide comfort and support in return. If your spouse isn't able to offer you the kind of support you need, be kind and patient, and if necessary, look for additional help from friends, family, or a therapist.

How can we, in times of emotional distance or alienation, rekindle emotional closeness and connection in our marriage?

Setting connection, vulnerability, and shared experiences as top priorities is necessary to rekindle emotional intimacy. Plan frequent dates or quality time spent together so that you may reconnect emotionally and concentrate on each other. Engage in empathy and active listening by focusing solely on each other's emotions and experiences. To promote a higher level of emotional understanding and connection, be open and honest about your feelings and vulnerabilities. Take part in routines or activities that deepen your relationship and help you make memories as a couple.

What are some practical ways for us to express our emotional needs to one another in a way that promotes empathy and support?

Emotional needs must be communicated clearly, vulnerable, and via active listening. Start by recognizing and expressing your own emotional needs and being transparent about what you want from your relationship. To communicate your thoughts and feelings without placing blame or offering criticism, use "I" statements. Recognize your partner's feelings and be willing to hear their point of view. In order to create a supportive environment where both partners feel heard and respected, practice empathy and make an effort to comprehend one other's emotional worlds.

Chapter Four

Decision-making in the presence of emotional trials

What steps should we take when one partner needs more emotional assistance due to mental health problems?

Helping a spouse who is struggling with mental health concerns calls for understanding, knowledge, and expert advice. Start by learning as much as you can about your partner's illness and how it impacts their feelings and actions. Urge your significant other to get professional assistance from a psychotherapist or anexperienced personnel who can offer them the direction and support they require. As your partner travels through their mental health journey, show them your unwavering love and support and show them that you are patient and understanding.

As we deal with the rigours and difficulties of daily life, how can we preserve emotional closeness and connection in our marriage?

Setting priorities, talking, and spending quality time together are all necessary to maintain an emotional connection. Schedule regular check-ins so that you can speak to each other about your thoughts, feelings, and experiences. Make date nights, shared hobbies, or private chats a priority. These activities foster intimacy and connection. Acts of kindness, encouraging words, and loving gestures are great ways to express your gratitude and love for your partner. Recall that creating a solid and happy marriage requires fostering emotional closeness.

What steps do we take when one partner's mental difficulties or past traumas affect our marriage's dynamics?

Managing emotional difficulties or traumas calls for tolerance, compassion, and, if necessary, expert assistance. Recognize that your spouse might be navigating challenging feelings or experiences as you approach the matter with compassion and understanding. If your partner's emotional problems are affecting their well-being and your relationship, encourage them to get professional assistance or therapy. As your partner works through their feelings, be patient and offer your support and assurance. Make an effort to provide a secure and encouraging atmosphere where your spouse feels appreciated and welcomed.

How can we negotiate variations in our coping mechanisms or emotional expression in a way that promotes acceptance and understanding amongst ourselves?

Empathy, inquiry, and compromise are necessary for navigating disparities in emotional expression. Realize that each person processes and expresses emotions in a way that is specific to them, influenced by their personality, experiences, and upbringing. Be curious about the problem and open to learning about each other's emotional lives. Seek a middle ground that honours the emotional needs and preferences of both partners while remaining receptive to compromise. Instead of attempting to alter one another's differences, focus on helping one another through them and exercising patience and acceptance.

In our marriage, how can we generate an environment where both partners feel free to express their most friendly thoughts and anxieties?

Establishing a secure and supportive atmosphere where both partners feel appreciated and accepted is essential to fostering emotional support and vulnerability. Engage in empathy and attentive listening, delving into one another's emotions and experiences without passing judgment. Promote openness and vulnerability by being honest about your feelings and worries, setting an example for your partner to follow. By acknowledging and respecting each other's weaknesses, you may foster trust and acceptance in your relationship. Honour times of emotional closeness and bonding by highlighting the value of communication and support in your union.

How do we respond when outside pressures or difficulties affect our capacity to offer each other emotional support?

Resilience, collaboration, and teamwork are necessary for managing external stressors. Understand that outside stressors like financial hardships, job demands, or health issues may affect your capacity to support one another emotionally. Given that the stressors may have varying effects on each partner, approach the situation with compassion and understanding. Be honest with each other about your thoughts and feelings, and collaborate to find workable solutions and coping mechanisms that will help you both feel less stressed and support one another during trying times.

What are some telltale signals that our marital emotional difficulties might require professional assistance or therapy?

Persistent feelings of melancholy, anxiety, or hopelessness; frequent arguments or breakdowns in communication that negatively affect your relationship; unresolved trauma or past experiences that still have an impact on your emotional well-being; and trouble handling stress or adjusting to significant life changes are all indicators that you may need professional assistance or therapy. Looking for support from a licensed therapist or counsellor may be helpful if you or your spouse are exhibiting any of these symptoms. They may offer direction and strategies to help you overcome your emotional obstacles and improve your relationship.

Chapter Five

Securing your relationship from external influence

In the face of significant life transitions like losing our jobs, moving, or losing a loved one, how can we assist one another emotionally?

Responding to each other's life transitions requires understanding, compassion, and flexibility. Show your spouse that you are there for them by paying attention to their worries and providing them with your undying support and assurance. Acknowledge and validate their emotions and sentiments, and when appropriate, offer helpful support in the form of tasks or scheduling. Be tolerant and empathetic, and exercise patience and adaptability as you work as a team to overcome the obstacles.

How can we help each other emotionally while facing significant life changes or obstacles, such as becoming parents, changing careers, or losing a loved one?

Collaboration, empathy, and communication are necessary for helping one another through changes. As a team, approach the situation and cooperate to overcome the obstacles and unknowns. Engage in active listening and offer nonjudgmental validation for each other's emotions and experiences. In order to reduce tension and demonstrate your dedication to one another, provide both practical and emotional support. Seek out tools and networks of support that can assist you both in overcoming the obstacles and changes productively.

How can we make sure that, even in the face of external stress or conflict, our emotional support for one another is steady and robust?

Setting priorities, being resilient, and being transparent are necessary to provide emotional support consistently. Even in times of outward stress or conflict, resolve to put your relationship and emotional connection first. To make sure you're in a healthy enough state to provide emotional support to your partner, engage in self-care and stress reduction practices. Openly discuss your needs and worries with one another, and even in the midst of difficulties, be there to encourage and understand one another. Keep in mind that your marriage's foundation is your emotional support for one another, which takes constant work and dedication to maintain.

How can we resolve conflicts between our emotional demands and other facets of our lives, such as family obligations or professional aspirations?

Empathy, dialogue, and compromise are necessary for resolving disputes involving emotional needs. Commence by candidly addressing the competing demands and worries, accepting one another's viewpoints and emotions without passing judgment. Make an effort to comprehend the guiding principles and reasons behind each partner's needs. Work together to come up with original ideas that, to the greatest extent feasible, meet the needs of both parties while also acknowledging that sometimes compromise is required. Put mutual respect and open communication first as you work through the challenges of striking a balance between your emotional needs and other responsibilities.

How can we help each other emotionally while facing significant life changes or obstacles, such as becoming parents, changing careers, or losing a loved one?

Collaboration, empathy, and communication are necessary for helping one another through changes. As a team, approach the situation and cooperate to overcome the obstacles and unknowns. Engage in active listening and offer nonjudgmental validation for each other's emotions and experiences. In order to reduce tension and demonstrate your dedication to one another, provide both practical and emotional support. Seek out tools and networks of support that can assist you both in overcoming the obstacles and changes productively.

About the Author

ADEGBOYE S. ADURAGBEMI is a manager, business administrator, entrepreneur, and motivational speaker in Africa. ADEGBOYE has his BA from Yale University, IPMA from Adonai University, and a Master's in Business Administration (MBA) from the University of Salford, Manchester.

He was born in South Africa but is presently based in Nigeria as a motivational speaker and marriage counsellor in institutions, sectors, and seminars with young and upcoming managers all over Africa.

Acknowledgements

I want to express my sincere gratitude to everyone who helped with the "FAQ on Communication in Marriage." Throughout this journey, their encouragement, insight, and support have been priceless.

I want to start by acknowledging the fact that, without God, this guide wouldn't have been possibly achieved.

And also, to my spouse, who has always been motivating and supportive in making this task successful, I will always love and appreciate you.

I have many couples to appreciate who have shared their experiences, challenges, and victories with me over the years. Your openness, weakness, and tenacity have enhanced the book's pages and provided priceless insights into the difficulties of marriage communication.

My sincere gratitude goes out to my family and friends for their continuous support and encouragement during this journey. Your wise advice, tolerance, and words of support have helped me get through the complicated process of writing and releasing this book.

I sincerely thank the specialists and experts who have so kindly offered their knowledge and skills in marriage and communication. Your advice and thoughts have improved this book's quality and depth, and I really appreciate your contributions.

Finally, I would like to express my profound gratitude to all of the readers of this work. As you journey through the process of communication in your marriage, I hope that the knowledge, direction, and encouragement provided within these pages will be a source of inspiration and empowerment for you. I sincerely appreciate your help.

www.ingramcontent.com/pod-product-compliance
Lightning Source LLC
Chambersburg PA
CBHW051251120626
46547CB00014B/1898